Peter Koch Jen

INTEGRATION OF

GLOMERULAR AND TUBULAR FUNCTION

IN NORMAL AND DIABETIC RAT KIDNEYS

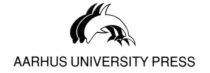

AARHUS UNIVERSITY PRESS

Typesetting: PC-Access ApS, Aarhus

Printed in Denmark by Werks Offset, Aarhus

ISBN 87 7288 273 5

AARHUS UNIVERSITY PRESS

Aarhus University

DK-8000 Aarhus C, Denmark

Denne afhandling er i forbindelse med på side iii nævnte tidligere publicerede arbejder af Det Lægevidenskabelige Fakultet ved Københavns Universitet antaget til offentligt at forsvares for den medicinske doktorgrad.

Københavns Universitet, den 18. maj 1989

Kjeld Møllgård

decanus

Forsvaret finder sted den 20. oktober 1989 kl. 14.00 præcis i anneksauditorium A, Studiegården, Studiestræde 6, København.

The present thesis is based on the following publications:

1. Jensen PK & K Steven. Angiotensin II induced reduction of peritubular capillary diameter in the rat kidney. Pflügers Archiv 371: 245-250, 1977.

2. Jensen PK & Steven K. Influence of intratubular pressure on proximal tubular compliance and capillary diameter in the rat kidney. Pflügers Archiv 382: 179-187, 1979.

3. Jensen PK, Christensen O & Steven K. A mathematical model of fluid transport in the kidney. Acta Physiol Scand 112: 373-385, 1981.

4. Jensen PK & Steven K. A model study of the tubuloglomerular feedback mechanism: effector site and influence on renal autoregulation. Acta Physiol Scand 115: 295-300, 1982.

5. Jensen PK, Christiansen JS, Steven K & Parving H-H. Renal function in streptozotocin-diabetic rats. Diabetologia 21: 409-414, 1981.

6. Jensen PK, Blæhr H & Steven K. Evaluation of the micropuncture determination of single nephron filtration fraction. Kidney Int 25: 486-491, 1984.

7. Jensen PK, Steven K, Blæhr H, Christiansen JS & Parving H-H. Effects of indomethacin on glomerular hemodynamics in experimental diabetes. Kidney Int 29: 490-495, 1986.

8. Jensen PK, Christiansen JS, Steven K & Parving H-H. Strict metabolic control and renal function in the streptozotocin diabetic rats. Kidney Int 31: 47-51, 1987.

CONTENTS

Acknowledgement

These experiments were undertaken during the tenure of a scholarship in 1976, and postdoctoral fellowships from 1979 to 1983 at the Department of General Physiology and Biophysics, The Panum Institute, Copenhagen University, Denmark.

I am deeply indebted to dr. med. Kenneth Steven for introducing me to the field of renal physiology. Without his never failing support and advice this study would not have been accomplished. I also owe tributes to prof. Hans Ulfendahl for teaching me the basics of micropuncture techniques. The implementation of digital computing techniques by lic. techn. Ove Christensen is highly appreciated. Prof. dr. med. Erik Skadhauge provided excellent laboratory facilities and support in times of trouble. The introduction to mathematical reasoning by prof. dr. med. Poul Kruhøffer and prof. dr. med. Ove Sten-Knudsen has been of great help. Also I am thankful to dr. med. Poul Peter Leyssac and prof. Don Marsh for many stimulating discussions on renal mathematical models. Prof. dr. med. Christian Crone and dr. med. Henrik Lund-Andersen are warmly thanked for creating an international atmosphere and attracting many excellent scientists to the Panum Institute. I am very grateful to dr. med. Jens Sandahl Christiansen, dr. med. Hans-Henrik Parving and especially dr. Barry Brenner for their introductions to the world of diabetic renal pathophysiology. The help of dr. Hanne Blæhr during part of the studies on the diabetic rats was indispensable.

The teaching of good craftsmanship by Kurt Juel-Sørensen, Hans Valdal and Svend Christoffersen is highly appreciated. Also Dorte Davidsen, Bodil Søndergaard, Nina Rasmussen and Bodil Aavad are thanked for good laboratory assistance.

Major economic support was provided by the funds of P. Carl Petersen, Johann and Hanne Weimann neé Seedorff, the Danish Medical Research Council, Steno Memorial Hospital, and "Landsforeningen for Sukkersyge". The studies were also supported by the foundations of Egmont H. Petersen, Hans Peter Poulsen and wife, Jacob Madsen and wife Olga Madsen, and the travelling fund of prof. August Krogh and dr. H. C. Hagedorn.

Finally the interest and support of my father during all phases of the study can never be adequately acknowledged.

Abbreviations

A   Afferent arteriolar index
AII   Angiotensin II
C   Plasma protein concentration
E   Efferent arteriolar index
GFR   Whole kidney glomerular filtration rate
GTB   Glomerulo-tubular balance
IDDM   Insulin dependent diabetes mellitus
K_F Glomerular ultrafiltration coefficient
NFF   Single nephron filtration fraction
NGFR   Single nephron GFR
P_{Bow} Bowman's space hydraulic pressure
P_G Glomerular capillary hydraulic pressure
ΔP Transmural glomerular capillary pressure (P_G - P_{Bow})
P_{Uf} Mean effective ultrafiltration pressure (NGFR / K_F)
RPF   Renal plasma flow rate
TGF   Tubuloglomerular feedback mechanism
π Plasma protein oncotic pressure

Introduction

Terrestrial life is dependent upon renal conservation of water and solutes. The excretion of waste products as urine is achieved by the production of a large quantity of glomerular ultrafiltrate (GFR) which is selectively reabsorbed by the tubular system. The glomerulo-tubular balance (GTB: the near constant ratio between GFR and the proximal tubular fluid reabsorption) is the intrinsic regulation that makes it possible to maintain the salt and water balance of the organism. Historically, alternating views on the causality of the interaction between glomerular and tubular function (Bojesen 1954, Kruhøffer 1960) have been advanced and reviewed (Leyssac 1976, Steven 1977): According to the "Copenhagen hypothesis" (Rehberg 1926) the tubular system possesses a considerable hydraulic resistance so that GFR cannot change significantly unless a primary change occurs in the rate of tubular fluid reabsorption. Alternatively GFR is determined by the ultrafiltration pressure in the glomerular capillaries and the proximal tubular reabsorption will follow GFR closely as a result of glomerulotubular balance maintained by several intrarenal mechanisms (Steven 1977, Ichikawa & Brenner 1980). The present study was performed to analyse the mechanism of GTB by quantifying the factors that determine the hydraulic resistance and the pressure in the tubular system.

GFR is increased during the early course of insulin-dependent diabetes mellitus (IDDM). This initial hyperfiltration is correlated to the late decrease in renal function which leads to renal insufficiency in a large fraction of the patients (Mogensen & Christensen 1984). Only the total rate of glomerular filtration (GFR) can be measured in patients. This is the integral of the function of all nephrons in the two kidneys. Alteration in GFR may be accomplished by a change in the number of functioning nephrons or in changes in the single nephron filtration rate (NGFR) (Brenner 1985). Measurement of NGFR and its determinants requires micropuncture of single nephrons, which up until now has only been carried out experimentally. In the second part of the thesis the determinants of NGFR are analysed in an animal model of IDDM.

Micropuncture methods

The present experiments were performed on Wistar rats anaesthetized with the barbiturates Inactin or Nembutal. In this rat strain no significant difference in tubular compliance was observed with these anaesthetics (Jensen & Steven 1979), but both agents caused a small decrease in renal function (Holstein-Rathlou et al. 1982), most likely as a result of their vasodepressant action. There is no a priori reason to expect different effects of these anaesthetics in diabetic and normal animals.

Streptozotocin was used to induce diabetes. This is a well known model with renal morphological counterparts (Hirose et al.1982) that resembles the changes observed in short term human insulin dependent diabetics (Kroustrup et al. 1977).

The preparation of the animals for micropuncture experiments required a free airway and intra-arterial and -venous lines for pressure measurements and fluid infusion. The kidney was immobilized in a lucite cup superfused with pre-warmed mineral oil to prevent drying. Superficial single nephrons and their adjoining vasculature were observed through a double-headed stereomicroscope permitting simultaneous micropuncture by two operators.

Pressure measurements in renal structures were performed actively by adjusting the pressure inside a glass micropipette to balance the outside pressure and prevent convective fluid movement at the tip. This was done either manually (Landis' technique) by inspecting the coloured interface or electronically (Wiederhielm's servo-nulling technique) by measurements of the resistance of 1M NaCl solution filling the pipette. Almost identical tubular pressures were recorded with the manual and the electronic systems (Jensen & Steven 1979). Precautions were taken to prevent artifacts in the electrical tip resistance measurements inside capillaries (Heyeraas-Tønder & Aukland 1979).

The glomerular capillary pressure was also measured indirectly by blocking the flow of tubular fluid in the early proximal tubule. The glomerular capillary pressure was then calculated as the sum of the stop flow tubular pressure and the plasma oncotic pressure. There are several theoretical objections to the use of this method but the results have been found to agree reasonably well with the direct method (Arendhorst & Gottschalk 1985). In our experiments the indirect method was found to overestimate the glomerular capillary pressure in normal Munich Wistar rats (Jensen & Kristensen 1985).

To allow calculations of the rate of tubular fluid reabsorption timed samples of tubular fluid were collected into oilfilled pipettes located in the last accessible segment of the proximal tubule or in the distal tubule. The pressure in the tubular system can be manipulated considerably by this pipette (Jensen & Steven 1979). Therefore it was monitored and care was taken to maintain the previously measured free flow value during the collection of tubular fluid (Jensen et al. 1981b, 1986, 1987).

Several methods were used for in vivo measurements of the dimensions of renal structures on photomicrographs of the renal surface. It was shown that it is possible to record absolute changes below the resolution of the microscope, which according to the Rayleigh criterion is the minimum distance between two separable points (Jensen & Steven 1977). Similar results for intratubular diameter were obtained by direct measurements on photomicrographs and calculation from the tubular pressure and flow rates (Jensen & Steven 1979).

Inulin was used to determine GFR. Albumin was used as a tracer of glomerular plasma flow since it is only ultrafiltered in negligible amounts (Jensen et al. 1984, 1987). Correct calculation of the single nephron filtration fraction (NFF) requires that the blood sample is representative of efferent glomerular blood which requires careful collection (Jensen et al. 1984). In addition to its convenience there is a theoretical advantage in using radioactive tracers which makes it possible to calculate NFF based upon the principle of mass conservation (Jensen et al. 1984). Most of the variance of the filtration fraction is caused by the radioactive counting statistics as a result of the small amount of tracers in the microsamples (Jensen et al. 1984). This is in contrast to the laborious alternate micromethod (Hughes & Ichikawa 1986) using measurements of protein concentration where replication on the same sample is possible, thereby permitting rejection of inconsistent values.

Internephron homogeneity is a prerequisite for renal micropuncture because efferent arteriolar blood sampling, tubular fluid sampling, and pressure measurements are performed in different nephrons. This seems to be fullfilled as the ratio of GFR to NGFR roughly equals the number of nephrons (Jensen et al. 1981b, 1986, and 1987). Furthermore, the glomerular capillary pressure is uniform in the rat kidney (Aukland et al. 1977). The superficial nephron filtration fraction is similar to the total kidney filtration fraction (Daugharty et al. 1972), notwithstanding that the value in the deepest nephrons may be different (Nissen 1966).

Tubular compliance

The distensibility of in vitro microdissected rabbit tubule is determined by its basement membrane (Welling & Grantham 1972). The response of the outer diameter of isolated rabbit proximal convoluted tubules to a change in pressure from 10 to 40 cmH_2O were recorded at 0.17 micron/cmH_2O (Welling & Grantham 1972) and 0.20 micron/cmH_2O (Pirie & Potts 1983), respectively, while the response of the inner diameter was found to be 0.39 micron/cmH_2O (Pirie & Potts 1983). It is not known whether the in vitro isolation procedure alters the elastic characteristics of the rabbit basement membrane. Similar proximal tubular compliance values have beeen measured in vivo in the anaesthetized rat (Cortell et al. 1973, Jensen & Steven 1979). Also, in diabetic rats the proximal tubules have similar distensibilities (Jensen et al. 1981c, Jensen unpublished).

It is conceivable that lower compliance values would have been recorded in the intact kidney where the tubules are packed closely together. One might expect that their distension would be constrained by the simultaneous expansion of all the tubules. This explanation appears unlikely because furosemide administration to the normal rat increased the intratubular pressure in all nephrons and the proximal and distal tubular diameter were observed to respond identically to the changes recorded in the partially obstructed single rat tubules in vivo (Cortell et al. 1973). Lower tubular compliances have been recorded in diuretic states induced by mannitol (Cortell et al. 1973) or 10% isotonic saline expansion (Sakai et al. 1986a), which are known to be associated with increased interstitial fluid pressure (Källskog & Wolgast 1973).

Proximal tubules and collecting ducts behave similarly to variations in the intratubular pressure with a decreased change in tubular diameter at increased pressure. This is the result of the non linear elastic properties of biological materials revealing a higher Young's modulus at increasing strain (Fung et al. 1966). In accordance with the experiments on isolated tubules (Pirie & Potts 1983) the proximal tubules in the intact kidney were found to be collapsible with a substantial higher compliance at low intratubular pressure (Jensen & Steven 1979).

It has been suggested that anaesthetics alter the tubular compliance (Elmer et al. 1973, Steven 1974). A priori it seems unlikely that the elastic constant of the basement membrane would be altered by anaesthesia. Accordingly, no differences in tubular compliances were obtained with two commonly employed barbiturates, Inactin and Nembutal (Jensen & Steven 1979). In contrast, significantly lower values for proximal tubular compliance were observed in experiments using a mixture of halothane and nitrous oxide to induce anaesthesia (Leyssac et al. 1986). The intratubular pressure was similar to that recorded in the inactin anaesthetized rat, and surprisingly, so was the tubular diameter. It is not known whether the interstitial pressure is lower during halothane than barbiturate anaesthesia. Alternatively the difference in the compliance values may be related to the function of contractile elements in the proximal tubule (Rostgaard et al. 1972).

The distal tubules have higher compliance values than the proximal tubules as a result of their lower transmural pressure (Cortell et al. 1973). There is a near linear relationship using a power function between the tubular diameter and pressure with an exponent that has the same value in different tubular segments (Jensen et al. 1981a). The loop of Henle in the superficial nephron is not directly accessible for micropuncture, but similar pressure-diameter relationships have been found as in other tubular segments of the rabbit kidney in vitro (Welling & Welling 1978).

Tubular hydrodynamics

The tubular system constitutes a considerable hydraulic resistance to axial fluid flow (Rehberg 1926, Kruhøffer 1960, Bojesen 1954, Leyssac 1976, Steven 1977). The proximal tubular pressure is relatively constant despite very large variations in the urine flow (Gottschalk & Mylle 1954). Consequently, tubular hydraulic resistance must be regulated. The confluence of the collecting ducts predominates over the fractional tubular fluid reabsorption by an order of magnitude (Jensen et al. 1981a) so that most of the resistance is located at the distal extreme of the tubular system (Marsh & Martin 1975, Steven 1977, Jensen et al. 1981a). Another significant part of the resistance is located in the loop of Henle as a result of its small diameter and considerable flow rate. Consequently, the segments comprising the major part of tubular resistance are located in the medulla. The implications of this fact and its relation to pelvic peristalsis remains unknown. The periodic flow in the collecting ducts caused by papillary milking (Jensen 1979, Reinking & Schmidt-Nielsen 1981) is very unlikely to change the pressure in the upstream tubular segments: A decrease in intratubular pressure will result in a decrease of diameter so that the collecting ducts will behave like a Starling resistor (Jensen & Steven 1979). This effect would be most pronounced distally where the tubular compliance is highest. In accordance, pressure oscillations synchronously with the pelvic contractions have never been observed in the proximal tubule (Holstein-Rathlou 1987) or in the distal tubule (Jensen, unpublished). Therefore, necrotic loss of the papillary tip is not likely to disturb glomerulo-tubular balance. On the other hand, during increased urine output where the largest relative increase in tubular flow rate occur in the collecting ducts, the milking activity of the papilla will propel the excessive fluid through the collecting duct system thereby creating a waterfall mechanism which eliminates the high terminal tubular hydraulic resistance. Hence, the reference pressure for tubular fluid hydraulic resistance calculations should be chosen somewhere along the cortical collecting ducts.

The pressure gradient in small tubes can be calculated by Hagen-Poiseuille's law neglecting its inertial terms due to the low value of Reynold's number. Therefore, the following second order effects on pressure dissipation can be neglected (Blick & Stein 1972): Gradual changes in diameter along the tubular system, the tortuos course of the nephron, irregularities of the walls as a result of cell protrusion (Welling & Welling 1975) or the brush border (Basmadjian et al. 1980), entrance effects at tubular branches, and tubular reabsorption interfering with the laminar flow profile (Macey 1965). In contrast, the distensibility of the tubules will make the pressure-flow relationship highly non linear (Jensen & Steven 1979).

The mathematical model of tubular flow in the proximal tubule was therefore based upon a modification of Poiseuille's law to take account of tubular compliance. Knowing the hydraulic pressure gradient along the proximal tubule, it is possible to calculate the flow rate (Jensen & Steven 1979). Proximal tubular compliance can be calculated from the change in the pressure gradient after application of suction by a micropipette inside the tubule. This calculated proximal tubular compliance was similar to the directly measured value. The modification of Poiseuille's equation therefore appears to be valid (Jensen & Steven 1979). Also, in experiments on the exposed papilla (Jensen 1979) the tubular diameter exponent in Poiseuille's equation was calculated at 3.9 (SEM = 0.3, N = 10) based on simultaneously measured values of the collecting duct pressure, flow, and diameter (Jensen, unpublished). This value is indistinguishable from the theoretical value. Also, in isolated perfused loops of Henle close agreement between tubular dimensions measured directly and calculated indirectly by Poiseuille's equation was observed at each pressure level (Welling & Welling 1975).

The kidney was modeled mathematically as a network of connected compliant tubes capable of fluid reabsorption. The transport constants to account for flow dependent fluid reabsorption were evaluated from the literature (Jensen et al. 1981a). The biophysical events underlying flow dependence of the tubular fluid reabsorption process has been reviewed recently (Wright 1982). The divergent experimental results (Jensen et al. 1981a) may be explained by possible artifacts in the micropuncture experiments involving artificial perfusion of a single proximal tubule. The composition of the tubular perfusate seems important, and particularly the use of native tubular fluid is crucial (Häberle & Davis 1985), but contrasting results have been obtained using harvested tubular fluid where only slight flow dependence was observed in another study (Peterson et al. 1986). Furthermore, cannulation of the proximal tubule with several micropipettes induces local trauma that may influence the results. Very few experimentators have controlled the tubular pressure during microperfusion. This perfusion pressure markedly influences the tubular morphology (Maunsbach et al. 1987). Alteration of the intratubular pressure will give rise to a change in reabsorption as a result of the hydraulic permeability of the tubular wall (Persson et al. 1975). Increasing the tubular perfusion rate by suction in the distal end of the proximal tubule will decrease the tubular pressure and augment NGFR (Steven 1974a). The decrease of the pressure and increase of NGFR will change the rate of fluid reabsorption in opposite direction and thereby cancel each other. On the other hand changing the flow rate by a perfusion pipette at a proximal site tends to change the tubular flow rate and pressure in the same direction. In conclusion, the majority of experiments shows that the tubular reabsorption process is highly flow dependent, in particular at reduced flow rates and when the tubular perfusate originates from the glomerulus.

The hydraulic pressure in the tubules was calculated from the tubular dimensions and the flow rate in the various segments. The influence of the pressure in Bowman's space (P_{Bow}) on the rate of ultrafiltration was then calculated iteratively until the solution converged (Jensen et al. 1981a). Alterations of several independent variables were made and the effect compared to values obtained experimentally. At the control operating point a change in the input to the tubular system (NGFR) of 1 nl/min in all nephrons resulted in a change of 0.2 mmHg in PBow. This is similar to the value derived empirically from experimental studies in another model (Huss et al. 1975).

7

The results show that tubular compliance and the flow dependent fluid reabsorption contribute about equally to stabilize the proximal intratubular pressure during variations in GFR with the chosen values of the independent variables. The model predicts the behaviour of the kidney in a number of simulations (Jensen et al. 1981a), but it fails to predict the diuretic state after massive NaCl expansion where the pressure drop across the loop of Henle is minimal (Gottschalk & Mylle 1954, Cortell et al. 1973, Sakai et al. 1986a). This may be explained by a too low estimate for the compliance of the loop of Henle. The superficial Henle's loop is inaccessible to direct observations so the diameter must be calculated indirectly from Poiseuille's equation using published experiments of single loop perfusions (Schnermann 1968, Koh & Baines 1974). The loop is thereby found to respond passively to the transmural pressure in an identical manner as in vivo perfused loop of Henle segments (Jensen et al. 1981a). In contrast, compliance values an order of magnitude larger are calculated from the transition between control conditions and the state of massive diuresis (Sakai et al. 1986a). This must be caused by an active regulation of the hydraulic resistance in the loop of Henle: In the same study (Sakai et al. 1986a) the calculated compliances in the proximal and distal tubules are lower than the values measured in partial blockade studies (Cortell et al. 1973) as a result of the increase in the cortical interstitial pressure associated with massive saline diuresis (*vide supra*). Also, both in the diabetic (Jensen et al. 1981b, Jensen et al. 1987) and the hypertensive rat (Stumpe et al. 1970) diuresis is associated with a decreased pressure gradient along the loop of Henle. This could be explained by a decrease in medullary interstitial pressure associated with diuresis but this explanation appears very unlikely. Hence, in the transition from hydropenia to diuresis there appears to be an intrinsic regulation of the resistance of the loop of Henle in superficial nephrons that cannot be explained quantitatively by their passive compliant characteristics (Koh & Baines 1974).

Determinants of glomerular ultrafiltration

NGFR is determined by the driving pressure across the glomerular ultrafiltration membrane and the value of its ultrafiltration coefficient (K_F). The effective ultrafiltration pressure depends on i) the systemic plasma protein concentration determining the oncotic pressure (π), ii) the glomerular capillary flow of plasma which influences the protein concentration profile along the capillary, iii) the hydraulic pressure inside the glomerular capillary (P_G), and iv) the pressure in Bowman's space (P_{Bow}). K_F is the product of the surface area of the glomerular capillary tuft facing Bowman's space and its hydraulic permeability.

Mathematical modeling has been used extensively to predict the complex influence of these determinants on NGFR. The models are based upon the Starling capillary filtration equation using as integration variable either the plasma protein concentration (Deen et al. 1972, Marshall & Trowbridge 1974, Steven & Strøbæk 1974) or the idealized capillary length (Blantz et al. 1974, Huss et al. 1975, Källskog et al. 1974). Similar results are obtained by these models and the more complex network models (Oken et al. 1981, Lambert et al. 1982). The present glomerular ultrafiltration model is identical to the model used by Brenner (Deen et al. 1972) having the following assumptions: i) the glomerular capillary tuft can be represented by a single tube, ii) the axial drop in hydraulic pressure along the capillary is negligable, iii) the protein oncotic pressure (π) can be expressed as a second order polynomium of the protein concentration, iv) concentration polarization effects inside the capillary are negligable.

Fig. 1: Sensitivity coefficients (S) of the glomerular ultrafiltration rate to perturbations of its determinants (X): The arterial protein concentration (C_A), transcapillary hydraulic pressure difference (ΔP), the ultrafiltration coefficient (K_F), and the rate of afferent plasma flow (RPF). The efferent ultrafiltration pressure ($\Delta P - \pi_E$) is shown on the abscissa.

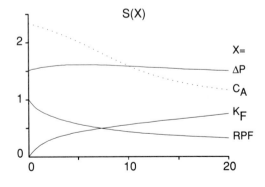

To test the mathematical model with experimental observations the glomerular capillary transmural pressure difference ($\Delta P = P_G - P_{Bow}$), NGFR and NFF are measured in different nephrons. Internephron variability is neglected in order to compile results for the calculation of the dependent variables. In addition, the following assumptions are made: i) the average pressures can be substituted for the pulsating pressures in the glomerular capillaries and in Bowman's space, ii) blood collected from the efferent arteriole is identical to that flowing out of the glomerular capillaries, iii) there is no correlation between the errors in the estimates of the dependent variables, iv) the calculation of K_F must be truncated when filtration equilibrium is attained to avoid the mathematical singularity when the denominator of the integral approaches zero (Jensen et al. 1986).

Much attention has been focused on the occurrence of filtration equilibrium *i.e.* the existence of a point along the glomerular capillary where π reaches ΔP, and consequently the filtration process terminates. To analyze the contribution of the determinants of GFR the sensitivity coefficients at various degrees of filtration equilibrium were calculated. The sensitivity coefficient S(X) is an indicator of the relative change in GFR for a given relative change in one determinant (X):

$$S(X) = \partial GFR / \partial X \cdot X / GFR$$

In the case where S(X) = 1 direct proportionality exists between GFR and X. The variables are thereby made dimensionless so they can be compared. Using the glomerulus model one of the determinants was changed by an infinitesimal amount leaving the remaining independent variables at their baseline values and the change in GFR was calculated. The degree of filtration equilibrium is given by the value of $\Delta P - \pi_E$ at the efferent end of the glomerular capillary. A range of paired K_F and ΔP values giving a baseline filtration fraction of 0.30 for an arterial plasma protein concentration of 57 g/l were calculated. The sensitivity coefficients were estimated for each pair. This analysis (Fig. 1) predicts that the oncotic and hydraulic pressures are the most important determinants of GFR only weakly influenced by the degree of filtration equilibrium. Conversely, the sensitivity of GFR to perturbations in K_F and the plasma flow are of lesser magnitude, but the degree of filtration equilibrium has a substantial influence on their sensitivity coefficients. These results are nearly identical when parameters corresponding to the human kidney are used *i.e.* a filtration fraction of 0.20 and a systemic plasma protein concentration of 70 g/l.

In contrast, based on extensive experimental evidence and analysis of covariance (Tucker & Blantz 1977), it is generally accepted that the plasma flow has a very strong influence on GFR and that the other determinants are of minor importance except in states far from filtration equilibrium. This may partly stem from the fact that plasma flow is calculated from GFR and the filtration fraction, raising the possibility of an artificial correlation (Riggs 1963): When two uncorrelated variables (x and y) vary randomly there will be a close correlation between one of the variables itself (x) and a derived function (y/x). Hence, suspicion should be raised whenever such correlations are presented and be accepted only if the measurement error of the determining variable is small compared to its total variance. However, such measures are rarely available in the literature.

Several regulatory systems contribute to the maintenance of GFR with the possibility of an offsetting effect whenever one of the determinants changes. The sensitivity coefficient of the mean effective ultrafiltration pressure (P_{Uf}) can be calculated at the expected value of 1.0 which is in contrast to the value of only 0.2 obtained experimentally (Arendhorst & Gottschalk 1985, fig. 4). This could be due to the demonstrated negative correlation between K_F and the ultrafiltration pressure. Mathematically K_F is given by NGFR/P_{Uf} raising the possibility of an artificial negative correlation between K_F and P_{Uf} (Riggs 1963). This is dependent on the ratio between the observed total variance of P_{Uf} and the variance due to its estimation. This is expected to be considerable as P_{Uf} is calculated from the glomerular capillary and Bowman's space pressures and the oncotic pressure integrated from the afferent to the efferent ends of the glomerular capillary. Thus, several components of the prediction error of P_{Uf} are present and its magnitude is only about 10 mmHg. The standard errors for individual animals are given in a study where P_{Uf} is changed by manipulating π in acute experiments (Tucker & Blantz 1981). These standard errors of P_{Uf} are surprisingly low compared to the standard errors of ΔP which can only be explained by some degree of crosscorrelation of the primary variables (Oken & Choi 1981). Thus, the prediction error of P_{Uf} is small compared to the observed change in P_{Uf} giving confidence to the conclusion that there is a real change in K_F. There is no morphologic counterpart to this phenomenon (Baylis et al. 1977). In isolated perfused dog glomeruli there is also a prominent effect of the perfusate protein concentration on K_F. These experiments have only been undertaken at normal and very low protein concentrations which has been found to increase K_F (Fried et al. 1986), possibly as a result of a direct effect on the capillary barrier (Michel et al. 1985).

To summarize: the glomerulus has been found to have the ability to regulate K_F in acute experiments when P_G or π is perturbated so making it possible to maintain NGFR constant. The mechamism is unknown. Several hormones have been shown to influence K_F (Baylis 1986), but the explanation awaits further experiments.

Effect of angiotensin II on renal capillaries

Angiotensin II (AII) is known to contract the renal vasculature and increase the filtration fraction mainly as a result of constriction of the efferent glomerular vessels *per se* (Myers et al. 1975, Ichikawa et al. 1979). The present results show that AII causes an active contraction of the peritubular capillaries when infused directly using a high physiological concentration (Jensen & Steven 1977). Most likely AII will also act on the efferent arteriole because this capillary network runs down in the renal parenchyma close to the ascending efferent arteriole (Jensen, unpublished microfill injections). Therefore, this method of infusing AII is a close approximation to its physiological release. These results can account for the increase in the glomerular capillary and proximal tubular pressures known to be associated with peritubular infusion

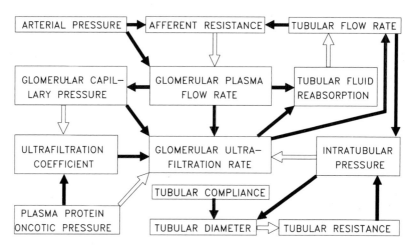

Fig 2. Feedback regulation scheme for the determinants of GFR. A filled or an open arrow between two variables indicates that the first variable increases or decreases the second variable, respectively. A loop with an even or odd number of open arrows constitutes a positive or negative feedback loop, respectively.

of AII (Steven 1974). In analogy, AII has been shown to decrease the glomerular diameter (Hornych et al. 1972) and it could thereby be involved by regulation of the capillary surface area available for filtration. Also, in isolated glomeruli AII decreases glomerular size (Sarschmidt et al. 1986), but no effect on the ultrafiltration coefficient (K_F) was found (Savin 1986). The glomerular contraction is thought to be accomplished by the mesangial cells (Kreisberg et al. 1982). The split hydronephrotic kidney shows no effect of topically applied AII on glomerular capillary diameter whereas a marked contraction is observed in the upstream arterioles and to a smaller extent in the efferent arteriole (Steinhausen et al. 1986). These models are unphysiologic since there is no flow in the tubular system. The same result, however, is obtained in intact kidneys where AII decreases glomerular size, but the capillary surface area is unchanged (Haley et al. 1987). It is possible that the reduction of K_F accomplished by physiological release of AII (Schor et al. 1981, Baylis 1986) is the result of mesangial contraction within the normal glomerulus and a decrease in the number of perfused capillaries. Alternatively, it is possible that the effect of AII on K_F is mediated by the increase in the glomerular capillary pressure per se (*vide supra*).

Regulation of GFR

Several intrarenal factors contribute to maintain the constancy of GFR as depicted in Fig. 2. These include the autoregulatory system that maintains RPF within a narrow range during changes in the arterial pressure by regulating the hydraulic resistance of the preglomerular arterioles (Heyeraas & Aukland 1987). The afferent arteriolar resistance is also increased by the macula densa negative feedback response (TGF) when the distal tubular flow rate or NaCl concentration rises above the normal level (Schnermann et al. 1970). In the deep nephrons the TGF response is also elicited when the flow rate is decreased (Sjöquist et al. 1984). The flow rate in the tubular system has a significant influence on the intratubular pressure which thereby exerts a negative feedback regulation of GFR (Rehberg 1926, Kruhøffer 1960). The intratubular pressure is also influenced by negative feedback of the tubular resistance resulting from its dependence on tubular diameter (Jensen & Steven 1979). The rate of tubular fluid reabsorption is dependent on the flow of ultrafiltrate into the early proximal tubule (Wright 1982) which exerts positive feedback regulation of GFR. This may also be accomplished by the peritubular plasma flow rate influencing the tubular reabsorption (Ichikawa & Brenner 1980). The rate of tubular reabsorption affects the flow past the macula densa cells (Jensen et al. 1982). The decrease in K_F associated with an increase in PG has been shown by experimental measurements but the mechanism remains unknown (*vide supra*).

The passive mechanisms are as powerfull as the TGF mechanism in stabilization of GFR (Jensen & Steven 1982). In the intact kidney simultaneous activation of TGF in all nephrons may amplify their effect by stimulating the interlobular arteries upstream from the afferent arterioles (Sjöquist et al. 1984). It has been shown that pressure oscillations in a nephron can be influenced by stimulation of its neighbours (Holstein-Rathlou 1987). Thus, the importance of the TGF mechanism for renal autoregulation in the intact kidney (Sakai et al. 1986b) might be larger than indicated by the gain calculated from perfusion experiments of individual nephrons (Jensen & Steven 1982, Briggs & Schnermann 1987, Aukland & Øien 1987).

Glomerular function in diabetes

Patients with insulin-dependent diabetes mellitus of recent onset (IDDM) have enlarged kidneys with increased GFR and filtration fraction. The renal plasma flow is only slightly increased. The arterial plasma protein concentration is similar to the value recorded in normal humans. The glomerular capillary pressure in humans cannot be measured directly. Most likely it is increased in diabetics: Assuming a normal afferent plasma flow, a baseline filtration fraction of 0.20, an arterial plasma protein concentration of 70 g/l, and ΔP similar to the value measured in normal dogs of 40 mmHg (Heller & Horacêk 1980), then the remaining determinant of GFR, K_F, can be calculated to have increased by 215% to account for the 20% increase in GFR. The same change in GFR could be accomplished by a 41% increase of K_F assuming ΔP to be 45 mm Hg. Therefore, the observed proportional increase in glomerular filtration surface and GFR in diabetics (Hirose et al. 1982) cannot be a causal relationship unless the K_F is very small in humans (and ΔP very high). This appears unlikely as isolated glomeruli from dogs and humans have similar K_F values (Savin 1981). Furthermore, the values of K_F measured in vitro (Savin 1981) agree closely with the values calculated in vivo from micropuncture data.

Moderately hyperglycemic rats with streptozotocin induced diabetes show the same relative increase of total renal function as observed in patients with short

14

term IDDM. The increase of GFR is to a small part caused by a decrease of the tubular resistance of unknown mechanism (Jensen et al. 1981b, 1987). The distensibility of the proximal tubules is known to be unchanged (Jensen et al. 1981c). The GTB is preserved in the diabetic rats (Jensen et al. 1981b, 1986, 1987). Hence, the rate of tubular fluid reabsorption cannot explain the increase of GFR since extreme alterations would be required to account for the observed hyperfiltration. By simple calculation (Fig. 1) this would require a substantial decrease of PBow and so causing reversal of the flow in the loop of Henle.

An increased glomerular transcapillary pressure has been demonstrated in the streptozotocin diabetic rat. Mathematical modelling (Jensen et al. 1987) shows that isomorphous growth of the renal structures does not give rise to increased glomerular capillary pressure. Hence, a decrease of the afferent/efferent ratio of the arteriolar resistance is required (Hostetter et al. 1981, Jensen et al. 1986, 1987).

Several hormonal systems may be involved in the increase of GFR in IDDM. In a recent review the effects of insulin, glucagon and growth hormone have been discussed (Christiansen 1985). AII, prostaglandins, vasopressin, and atrial natriuretic peptide all influence the determinants of GFR.

AII causes a rise in Puf and NFF and a decrease in K_F (Myers et al. 1975). The plasma renin activity in diabetic rats is decreased (Christlieb 1974) and the density of glomerular AII receptors are reduced (Ballerman et al. 1984). Accordingly, a decreased renal response has been found to systemically administered AII (Reineck & Kreisberg 1983). Also, cultured mesangial cells have been shown to require insulin in order to contract when exposed to AII (Kreisberg et al. 1982). A decreased contractile response to AII was observed in isolated glomeruli from diabetic rats (Kikkawa et al. 1986). Contrasting results have been obtained showing a normal AII response in diabetics (Barnett et al. 1987, Bank et al. 1988).

The role of the renal prostaglandins also appears controversial: No effect of prostaglandin inhibition on GFR was observed in one human study (Christiansen et al. 1985), but opposite results were obtained in another (Craven et al. 1987). No effect of Indomethacin or aprotinin on renal function were observed in rats with short duration of streptozotocin induced diabetes (Bank et al. 1988). These results are challenged by the findings in another rat study showing that chronic Indomethacin treatment prevents the initial hyperfiltration (Kirschenbaum & Chaudhari 1986). Three months after the induction of diabetes (Jensen et al. 1986) a very dramatic effect of Indomethacin was observed causing

15

normalization of PG. This finding is corroborated by observation of a substantial decrease of the degree of proteinuria in patients with nephropathy (Hommel et al. 1987). These apperantly contrasting results may be explained by variations in time in the concentration of the prostaglandins in early diabetes (Quilley & McGiff 1985). Usually the prostaglandin system is activated as a compensatory response to maintain glomerular function. Hence, prostaglandin activation is more likely to occur during the later phases of the disease. Clearly, more experiments are needed to clarify this point.

An increased vasopressin concentration has been found in diabetic rats (van Itallie et al. 1982), but the animals were not given insulin and the increased hormone concentration could be a result of dehydration. The kallikrein system has also been reported to be affected in diabetes but no consistent findings have been reported so far (Mayfield et al. 1984, 1985).

Atrial natriuretic peptide seems a most likely effector since it increases PG (Schnermann et al. 1986, Dunn et al. 1986) and its concentration has been found to be increased in diabetic rats (Ortola et al. 1987). Streptozotocin diabetic rats have increased blood and plasma volume (Hostetter et al. 1981, Jensen et al. 1986) which may explain the release of the atrial natriuretic hormone. An increased glomerular capillary pressure despite normal plasma volume also has been observed (Jensen et al. 1987).

The macula densa mediated TGF system is reset in the diabetic rats so permitting the rise of GFR (Jensen et al. 1986). The exact mechanism is unknown. It has been shown that glucose can decrease the TGF sensitivity in acute experiments (Blantz et al. 1982), although the associated increase in renal interstitial pressure caused by the volume expansion may also be involved. Several of the hormonal systems discussed above are known to change the TGF sensitivity (Briggs & Schnermann 1987). Consequently, the efficacy of renal autoregulation will be reduced so that transient changes in the arterial pressure will be transmitted to the glomerular capillaries.

The following theory for the pathogenesis of diabetic nephropathy has been proposed (Brenner 1985, Hostetter 1985): The increase in PG causes glomerular sclerosis that will decrease the number of active nephrons. This leads to a vicious cycle by imposing a further work load on the remaining functioning nephrons which in turn will result in a further rise in PG (Brenner et al. 1982). This theory is supported by experimental observations in the streptozotocin diabetic rat showing retardation of the development of glomerular sclerosis following normalization of PG, either by protein restriction or inhibition of the angiotensin converting enzyme (Zatz et al. 1985, 1986). The theory has been challenged recently (Bank et al. 1987), but the conclusion in this study is dependent on comparison between spontanously hypertensive and Wistar Kyoto rats. Apart from that particular comparison, these experiments show a very good relationship between P_G and the degree of glomerular sclerosis (Bank et al. 1987). Also, in systemic capillaries there is a correlation between the pressure and the basement membrane thickness (Williamson et al. 1971). Therefore, increasing ΔP may result in thickening of the basement membrane (Hirose et al. 1982). It may also be pertinent that a high intracapillary pressure is a common feature of the capillary beds in the organs that are most seriously affected by late diabetic manifestations: The glomerulus, the retina and the feet.

Direct proof of the hyperfiltration theory requires sequential micropuncture studies showing a correlation between the increase in P_G and the development of glomerular sclerosis. Such studies have recently been published failling to support the hypothesis (Yoshida et al. 1988). Furthermore, the focal glomerular sclerosis observed in the streptozotocin induced diabetic rat model is rarely seen in human diabetics. Conversely, rats do not develop the Kimmelstiel-Wilson lesion of the glomerulus. Therefore, this rat model may not be an ideal model of human diabetic nephropathy (Fine 1988, Steffes et al. 1982).

Summary

The present study was made to examine the validity of the Brandt-Rehberg hypothesis according to which the rate of glomerular ultrafiltration is almost entirely determined by the rate of tubular fluid reabsorption (absaugen). Micropuncture experiments were made to measure the influence of the hydraulic pressure on proximal tubular diameter and its axial pressure gradient. A tubular model was based upon Poiseuille's law taking into account the distensibility of the tubules. Also, the influence of luminal flow rate on the rate of tubular fluid reabsorption was evaluated. The results derived from this model were found to predict accurately the experimental observed pressure-flow relationship recorded in the single nephron. To analyse renal fluid transport a mathematical model of the glomerulus was coupled to the tubular model. The intratubular pressure was found to vary little, allowing the rate of glomerular filtratration rate to change as a result of alterations in the driving glomerular capillary pressure. The tubular flow rate was found to exert a powerful effect on GFR, mainly as a result of the macula densa mediated feedback regulation of the afferent arteriolar resistance. Also, the effective glomerular ultrafiltration coefficient is regulated by unknown mechanisms which stabilizes GFR.

The model was used to evaluate the mechanism of increased GFR in rats with experimentally induced diabetes. An increased glomerular capillary transmural pressure difference was the main cause of the rise in GFR. A close correlation was found between the increase in the filtration pressure and a decrease in the ultrafiltration coefficient. This may initiate a vicious cycle causing a further decrease in capillary permeability eventually leading to development of diabetic nephropathy. The experimental studies showed that peritubular capillaries are able to constrict actively in normal rats. This may explain angiotensin II mediated decrease in the hydraulic permeabiliy of the glomerular capillary membrane and the increased filtration fraction. This mechanism, however, does not appear to be responsible for the changes observed in experimental diabetes although treatment with angiotensin converting enzyme inhibition has a beneficial effect on the long term outcome. Recent experiments suggest that the atrial natriuretic peptide is responsible for the initial alteration of glomerular function in experimental diabetes. In addition, the prostaglandin system is known to be activated in the diabetic rats and inhibition by Indomethacin was found to normalize the glomerular capillary pressure. Furher experiments are needed to clarify whether this effect can be applicated therapeutically to preserve the renal function in diabetes.

Summary in Danish

Undersøgelsen blev udført for at analysere determinanterne af den glomerulære filtrationshastighed (GFR) på baggrund af Brandt-Rehberg's hypotese. Ifølge denne kan GFR ikke øges med mindre der sker en primær stigning i tubulusreabsorptionen, fordi det distale tubulus system besidder en væsentlig hydraulisk modstand under normale omstændigheder. Det påvises, at tubulus modstanden er dynamisk, idet det transmurale tryk påvirker tværsnitsdiameteren og dermed den aksiale hydrauliske modstand. Det intratubulære tryk er således reguleret ved en negativ tilbagekobling gennem distensibiliteten af tubulusvæggen. Denne regulationsmekanisme forstærkes af den tubulære flowafhængige væskereabsorption, der vil bevirke at kun en lille fraktion af en primær ændring i GFR udskilles som urin. Hypotesens præmisser er derfor ukorrekte. Koncentrationen af NaCl og flowhastigheden forbi cellerne i macula densa har en tonisk effekt på den afferente arterioles hydrauliske modstand og udøver dermed regulation af GFR ved negativ tilbagekobling. Hypotesens konklusion er derfor korrekt, idet en isoleret ændring af GFR kræver en omjustering af tilbagekoblingsmekanismen. Endvidere sker der et fald i den glomerulære ultrafiltrationskoefficient, når ultrafiltrationstrykket øges. Disse mekanismer bevirker at GFR holdes inden for snævre rammer under normale forhold.

Hos rotter med streptozotocin induceret sukkersyge påvistes de samme ændringer i GFR, som er blevet observeret hos patienter med nyopdaget insulin afhængig diabetes mellitus. Ved mikropunktur fandtes forhøjet tryk i de ultrafiltrerende hårkar og nedsat tryk i tubulussystemet på grund af reduceret modstand i Henle's slynge. Den glomerulo-tubulære balance fandtes bevaret hos diabetiske dyr. Årsagen til forøgelsen af GFR fandtes væsentligst at være forårsaget af det øgede glomerulære filtrationstryk. Dette var endvidere korreleret til nedsættelsen af hårkarrenes væskegennemtrængelighed. Denne mekanisme antages at være af central betydning for udviklingen af den sene manifestation af sygdommen med nyresvigt, idet en beskyttende effekt er observeret ved behandling og normalisering af trykket i hårkarrene efter indgift af angiotensin konverterende enzym hæmmer. I nærværende arbejde kunne normalisering af det øgede glomerulus kapillær tryk påvises efter hæmning af prostaglandin dannelsen med Indomethacin. Dette kunne i fremtidige studier underkastes en klinisk afprøvning af en mulig bevarende effekt på nyrefunktionen hos patienter med begyndende sendiabetiske manifestationer.

References

ARENDHORST, WJ & GOTTSCHALK, CW 1985. Glomerular ultrafiltration dynamics: historical perspective. Am J Physiol 248: F163-F175.

AUKLAND, K & ØIEN, AH 1987. Renal autoregulation models combining tubuloglomerular feedback and myogenic response. Am J Physiol 252: F768-F783.

AUKLAND, K, TØNDER, KH & NÆSS, G 1977. Capillary pressure in deep and superficial glomeruli of the rat kidney. Acta Physiol Scand 101: 418-427.

BALLERMANN, BJ, SKORECKI, KL & BRENNER, BM 1984. Reduced glomerular angiotensin II receptor density in early untreated diabetes mellitus in the rat. Am J Physiol 247: F110-F116.

BANK, N, AYNEDJIAN, HS, NGUYEN, D & SABLAY, LB 1987. Evidence against increased glomerular pressure initiating diabetic nephropathy. Kidney Int 31: 898-905.

BANK, N, LAHORRA, MAG, AYNEDJIAN, HS & SCHLONDORFF, D 1988. Vasoregulatory hormones and the hyperfiltration of diabetes. Am J Physiol 254: F202-F209.

BARNETT, R, SCHARSCHMIDT, L, YOUNG-HYEH, K & SCHLONDORFF, D 1987. Comparison of glomerular and mesangial prostaglandin synthesis and glomerular contraction in two rat models of diabetes mellitus. Diabetes 36: 1468-1475.

BASMADJIAN, DS, DYKES, DS & BAINES, AD 1980. Flow through brushborders and similar protuberant wall structures. J Memb Biol 56: 183-190.

BAYLIS, C 1986. Glomerular filtration dynamics. In: Advances in Renal Physiology. Editor Lote. Croom & Helm.

BAYLIS, C, ICHIKAWA, I, WILLIS, WT, WILSON, CB & BRENNER, BM 1977. Dynamics of glomerular ultrafiltration IX. Effects of plasma protein concentration. Am J Physiol 232: F58-F71.

BLANTZ, RC 1974. Effect of mannitol on glomerular ultrafiltration in the hydropenic rat. J Clin Invest 54: 1135-1143.

BLANTZ, RC, PETERSON, ÖW, GUSHWA, L & TUCKER, BJ 1982. Effect of modest hyperglycemia on tubuloglomerular feedback activity. Kidney Int 22: S206-S212.

BLICK, EF & STEIN, PD 1972. A review of second-order effects on Poiseuille's equation for application to blood and other viscous fluids. Med Res Engn 11: 27-34.

BOJESEN, E 1954. The renal mechanism of "dilution diuresis" and salt excretion in dogs. Acta Physiol Scand 32: 129-147.

BRENNER, BM 1985. Nephron adaptation to renal injury or ablation. Am J Physiol 249: F324-337.

BRENNER, BM, MEYER, TW & HOSTETTER, TH 1982. Dietary protein intake and the progressive nature of kidney disease: The role of hemodynamically mediated glomerular injury in the pathogenesis of progressive glomerular sclerosis in aging, renal ablation, and intrinsic renal disease. New Engl J Med 307: 652-659.

BRIGGS, JP & SCHNERMANN, J 1987. The tubuloglomerular feedback mechanism. Ann Rev Physiol 49: 251-273.

CHRISTIANSEN, JS 1985. Glomerular hyperfiltration in diabetes mellitus. Diabetic Medicine 2: 235-239.

CHRISTIANSEN, JS, RASMUSSEN, JF & PARVING, H-H 1985. Short-term inhibition of prostaglandin synthesis has no effect on the elevated glomerular filtration rate of early insulin-dependent diabetes. Diabetic Medicine 2:17-20.

CHRISTLIEB, AR 1974. Renin, angiotensin, and norepinephrine in alloxan diabetes. Diabetes 23: 962-970.

CORTELL, S, GENNARI, FJ, DAVIDMAN, M, BOSSERT, WH & SCHWARTZ, WB 1973. A definition of proximal and distal tubular compliance. J Clin Invest 52: 2330-2339.

CRAVEN, PA, CAINES, MA & DERUBERTIS, FR 1987. Sequential alterations in glomerular prostaglandin and thromboxane synthesis in diabetic rats: Relationship to the hyperfiltration of early diabetes. Metabolism 36: 95-103.

DAUGHARTY, TM, UEKI, IF, NICHOLAS, DP & BRENNER, BM 1972. Comparative renal effects of isoncotic and colloid-free volume expansion in the rat. Am J Physiol 222: 225-235.

DEEN, WM, ROBERTSON, CR & BRENNER, BM 1972. A model of glomerular ultrafiltration in the rat. Am J Physiol 223: 1178-1183.

DUNN, BR, ICHIKAWA, I, PFEFFER, J, TROY, JL & BRENNER, BM 1986. Renal and systemic hemodynamic effects of synthetic atrial natriuretic peptide in the anesthetized rat. Circ Res 59: 237-246.

ELLIS, EN, STEFFES, MW, GOETZ, FC, SUTHERLAND, DER & MAUER, SM 1986. Glomerular filtration surface in type I diabetes mellitus. Kidney Int 29: 889-894.

ELMER, M, KRISTENSEN, LØ & LEYSSAC, PP 1973. Proximal luminal diameters and cell volume in rats anesthetized with inactin and amytal. Acta Physiol Scand 88: 226-233.

FINE, LG 1988. Preventing the progression of human renal disease: Have rational therapeutic principles emerged? Kidney Int 33: 116-128.

FRIED, TA, MCCOY, RN, OSGOOD, RW & STEIN, JH 1986. Effect of albumin on glomerular ultrafiltration coefficient in isolated perfused dog glomerulus. Am J Physiol 250: F901-F906.

FUNG, YC, ZWEIFACH, BW & INTAGLIETTA, M 1966. Elastic environment of the capillary bed. Circ Res 19: 441-461.

GOTTSCHALK, CW & MYLLE, M 1957. Micropuncture study of pressure in proximal and distal tubules and peritubular capillaries of the rat kidney during osmotic diuresis. Am J Physiol 189: 323-328.

HALEY, DP, SARRAFIAN, M BULGER, RE, DOBYAN, DC & EKNOYAN, G 1987. Structural and functional correlates of effects of angiotensin induced changes in rat glomerulus. Am J Physiol 253: F111-F119; 1987.

HELLER, J & HORACÊK, V 1980. Comparison of directly measured and calculated glomerular capillary pressure in the dog kidney at varying perfusion pressure. Pflügers Arch 385: 253-258.

HEYERAAS TØNDER, K & AUKLAND, K 1979. Glomerular capillary pressure in the rat. Acta Physiol Scand 109: 93-95.

HEYERAAS, K J & AUKLAND, K 1987. Interlobular arterial resistance: Influence of renal arterial pressure and angiotensin II. Kidney Int 31: 1291 - 1298.

HIROSE, K, ØSTERBY, R, NOZAWA, M & GUNDERSEN, HJG 1982. Development of glomerular lesions in experimental long-term diabetes in the rat. Kidney Int 21: 689-695.

HOLSTEIN-RATHLOU, NH 1987. Synchronization of proximal intratubular pressure oscillations: evidence for interaction between nephrons. Pflügers Arch 408: 438-443.

HOLSTEIN-RATHLOU, NH, CHRISTENSEN, P & LEYSSAC, PP 1982. Effects of halothane-nitrous oxide inhalation anaesthesia and inactin on overall renal function in Sprague-Dawley and Wistar rats. Acta Physiol Scand 114: 193-201.

HOMMEL, E, MATHIESEN, E, ARNOLD-LARSEN, S, EDSBERG, B, OLSEN, UB & PARVING, H-H 1987. Effects of indomethacin on kidney function in type I (insulin-dependent) diabetic patients with nephropathy. Diabetologia 30: 30.

HORNYCH, H, BEAUFILS, M & RICHET, G 1972. The effect of exogenous angiotensin on superficial and deep glomeruli in the rat kidney. Kidney Int 2: 336-343.

HOSTETTER, TH 1985. Diabetic nephropathy. New Engl J Med 312: 642-643.

HOSTETTER, TH, TROY, JL & BRENNER, BM 1981. Glomerular hemodynamics in experimental diabetes mellitus. Kidney Int 19: 410-415.

HUGHES, ML & ICHIKAWA, I 1986. Interglomerular heterogeneity of filtration fraction among superficial nephrons. Kidney Int 29: 814 - 819.

HUSS, RE, MARSH, DJ & KALABA, RE 1975. Two models of glomerular filtration rate and renal blood flow in the rat. Ann Biomed Engn 3: 72-99.

HÄBERLE, DA & VON BAYER, H 1983. Characteristics of glomerulotubular balance. Am J Physiol 244: F355-F365.

ICHIKAWA, I & BRENNER, BM 1980. Importance of efferent arteriolar vascular tone in regulation of proximal tubule fluid reabsorption and glomerulotubular balance in the rat. J Clin Invest 65: 1192-1201.

ICHIKAWA, I, MIELE, JF & BRENNER, BM 1979. Reversal of renal cortical actions of angiotensin II by verapamil and manganese. Kidney Int 16: 137-147.

JENSEN, PK 1979. Continuous measurement of flow rate and volume in the nanoliter range. Acta Physiol Scand 106: 5-9.

JENSEN, PK & KRISTENSEN, KS 1985. Glomerular capillary pressure in diabetic rats. Acta Physiol Scand 124 suppl 542: 196.

JENSEN, PK & STEVEN, K 1977. Angiotensin II induced reduction of peritubular capillary diameter in the rat kidney. Pflügers Archiv 371: 245-250.

JENSEN, PK & STEVEN, K 1979. Influence of intratubular pressure and anaesthesia on proximal tubular compliance and capillary diameter in the rat kidney. Pflügers Archiv 382: 179-187.

JENSEN, PK & STEVEN, K 1982. Tubuloglomerular feedback mechanism: A model study of the effector site and influence on renal autoregulation. Acta Physiol Scand 115: 295-300.

JENSEN, PK, BLÆHR, H & STEVEN, K 1984. Evaluation of the micropuncture determination of single nephron filtration fraction. Kidney Int 25: 486-491.

JENSEN, PK, CHRISTENSEN, O & STEVEN, K 1981a. A mathematical model of fluid transport in the nephron. Acta Physiol Scand 112: 373-385.

JENSEN, PK, CHRISTIANSEN, JS, STEVEN, K & PARVING, H-H 1981b. Renal function in streptozotocin diabetic rats. Diabetologia 21: 409-415.

JENSEN, PK, CHRISTIANSEN, JS, STEVEN, K & PARVING, H-H 1981c. Renal function in diabetic rats. Acta Endocrin 97 suppl 242: 25.

JENSEN, PK, KRISTENSEN, KS, RASCH, R & PERSSON, EAG 1986. Resetting of the tubuloglomerular feedback mechanism in diabetic rats. Acta Endocrin 112 suppl. 275: 12.

JENSEN, PK, STEVEN, K, BLÆEHR, H, CHRISTIANSEN, JS & PARVING, H-H 1986. The effects of indomethacin on glomerular hemodynamics in experimental diabetes. Kidney Int 29: 490-495.

JENSEN, PK, CHRISTIANSEN, JS, STEVEN, K & PARVING, H-H 1987. Strict metabolic control and renal function in the streptozotocin diabetic rat. Kidney Int 31: 47-51.

KASISKE, BL, O'DONNELL, MP & KEANE, WF 1985. Glucose-induced increases in renal hemodynamic function. Possible modulation by renal prostaglandins. Diabetes 34: 360-364.

KIKKAWA, R, KITAMURA, E, FUJIWARA, Y, ARIMURA, T, HANEDA, M & SHIGETA, Y 1986. Impaired contractile responsiveness of diabetic glomeruli to angiotensin II: A possible indication of mesangial dysfunction in diabetes mellitus. Biochem Biophys Res Comm 136: 1185-1190.

KIRSCHENBAUM, MA & CHAUDHARI, A 1986. Effect of experimental diabetes on glomerular filtration rate and glomerular prostanoid production in the rat. Mineral Electrol Metab 12: 352-355.

KOH, YG & BAINES, AD 1974. Pressure-flow relationships in Henle's loops and long collapsible rubber tubes. Kidney Int 5: 30-38.

KREISBERG, JI 1982. Insulin requirement for contraction of cultured rat glomerular mesangial cells in response to angiotensin II: Possible role for insulin in modulating glomerular hemodynamics. Proc Natl Acad Sci 79: 4190-4192.

KROUSTRUP, JP, GUNDERSEN, HJG & ØSTERBY, R 1977. Glomerular size and structure in diabetes mellitus. III. Early enlargement of the capillary surface. Diabetologia 13: 207-210.

KRUHØFFER, P 1960. Handling of alkali metal ions by the kidney. In: The alkali metal ions in biology. Eds. Ussing, H, Kruhøffer, P, Hess-Thaysen, J and NA Thorn. Berlin, Göttingen, Heidelberg: Springer Verlag IV.C: 261-268.

KÄLLSKOG, Ö & WOLGAST, M 1973. Driving forces over the peritubular capillary membrane in the rat kidney during antidiuresis and saline expansion. Acta Physiol Scand 89: 116-125.

KÄLLSKOG, Ö, LINDBOM, LO, ULFENDAHL, HR & WOLGAST, M 1975. Kinetics of glomeurlar ultrafiltration in the rat kidney. A theoretical study. Acta Physiol Scand 95: 191-200.

LAMBERT, PP, AEIKENS, B, BOHLE, A, HANUS, F, PEGOFF, S & VANDAMME, M 1982. A network model of glomerular function. Microvasc Res 23: 99-128.

LEYSSAC, P 1976. The renin angiotensin system and kidney function. A review of contributions to a new theory. Acta Physiol Scand suppl 442: 1-52.

LEYSSAC, PP, JENSEN, PK & HOLSTEIN-RATHLOU, N 1986. A study of proximal tubular compliances in normotensive and spontaneously hypertensive rats, and the effect of anaesthesia on the compliance. Acta Pysiol Scand 126: 341-348.

MACEY, RI 1965. Hydrodynamics in the renal tubule. Bull Math Biophysics 27: 117-124.

MARSHALL, EA & TROWBRIDGE, EA 1974. A mathematical model of the ultrafiltration process in a single glomerular capillary. J Theor Biol 48: 389-412.

MARSH, DJ & MARTIN, CM 1975. Effects of diuretic states on collecting duct fluid flow resistance in the hamster kidney. Am J Physiol 229: 13-17.

MAUNSBACH, AB, GIEBISCH, GH & STANTON, BA 1987. Effects of flow rate on proximal ultrastructure. Am J Physiol 253: F582-F587.

MAYFIELD, RK, MARGOLIUS, HS, LEVINE, JH, WOHLTMANN, HJ, LOADHOLT, CB & COLWELL, JA 1984. Urinary kallikrein excretion in insulin-dependent diabetes mellitus and its relationship to glycemic control. J Clin Endocrin Metab 59: 278-286.

MAYFIELD, RK, MARGOLIUS, HS, BAILEY, GS, MILLER, DH, SENS, DA, SQUIRES, J & NAMM, DH 1985. Urinary and renal tissue kallikrein in the streptozotocin-diabetic rat. Diabetes 34: 22-28.

MICHEL, CC, PHILLIPS, ME & TURNER, MR 1985. The effects of native and modified bovine serum albumin on the permeability of frog mesenteric capillaries. J Physiol 360: 333-346.

MOGENSEN, CE & CHRISTENSEN, CK 1984. Predicting diabetic nephropathy in insulin-dependent patients. N Engl J Med 311: 89-93.

MYERS, BD, DEEN, WM & BRENNER, BM 1975. Effects of norepinephrine and angiotensin II onh the determinants of glomerular ultrafiltration and proximal tubule fluid reabsorption in the rat. Circ Res 37: 101-110.

NISSEN, OI 1966. Filtration fractions of plasma supplying the superficial and deep venous drainage area of the cat kidney. Acta Physiol Scand 68: 275-285.

OKEN, DE & CHOI, SC 1981. Filtration pressure equilibrium: A statistical analysis. Am J Physiol 241: F196-F200.

OKEN, DE, THOMAS, SR & MIKULECKY, DC 1981. A network thermodynamic model of glomerular dynamics: Application in the rat. Kidney Int 19: 359-373.

ORTOLA, FV, BALLERMAN, BJ, ANDERSON, S & BRENNER, BM 1987. Elevated atrial natriuretic peptide levels in diabetic rats. J Clin Invest 80: 670-674.

PETERSON, ÖW, GUSHWA, LC & BLANTZ, RC 1986. An analysis of glomerulotubular balance. Pflügers Arch 407: 221-227.

PERSSON, AEG, SCHNERMANN, J, ÅGERUP, B ERIKSSON, NE 1975. The hydraulic conductivity of the rat poximal tubular wall determined with colloidal solutions. Pflügers Arch 360: 25-44.

PIRIE, SC & POTTS, DJ 1983. The effect of peritubular protein upon fluid reabsorption in rabbit proximal convoluted tubules perfused in vitro. J Physiol 337: 429-440.

QUILLEY, J & MCGIFF, JC 1985. Arachidonic acid metabolism and urinary excretion of prostaglandins and thromboxane in rats with experimental diabetes mellitus. J Pharm Exp Therap 234: 211-216.

REHBERG, PB 1926. The rate of filtration and reabsorption in the human kidney. Biochem J 20: 447-460.

REINECK, HJ & KREISBERG, JI 1983. Renal vascular response to angiotensin II in rats with streptozotocin-induced diabetes mellitus. Kidney Int 23: 247.

REINKING, LN & SCHMIDT-NIELSEN, B 1981. Peristaltic flow of urine in the renal papillary collecting ducts of hamsters. Kidney Int 20: 55-60.

RIGGS, DS 1963. The mathematical approach to physiological problems. Williams & Wilkins. Baltimore

ROSTGAARD, J, KRISTENSEN, BI & NIELSEN, LE 1972. Electron microscopy of filaments in the basel part of rat kidney tubule cells, and their in situ interaction with heavy meromyuosin. Z Zellforsch 132: 497-521.

SAKAI, T, CRAIG, DA, WEXLER, AS & MARSH, DJ 1986a. Fluid waves in renal tubules. Biophys J 50: 805-813.

SAKAI, T, HALLMAN, E & MARSH, DJ 1986b. Frequency domain analysis of renal autoregulation in the rat. Am J Physiol 250: 364-373.

SAVIN, VJ 1986. In vitro effects of angiotensin II on glomerular function. Am J Physiol 251: F627-F634.

SAVIN, VJ & TERREROS, DA 1981. Filtration in single isolated mammalian glomeruli. Kidney Int 20: 188-197.

SCHARSCHMIDT, LA, DOUGLAS, JG & DUNN, MJ 1986. Angiotensin II and eicosanoids in the control of glomerular size in the rat and human. Am J Physiol 250: F348-F356.

SCHNERMANN, J, MARIN-GREZ, M & BRIGGS, JP 1986. Filtration pressure response to infusion of atrial natriuretic peptides. Pflügers Arch 406: 237-239.

SCHNERMANN, J 1968. Microperfusion study of single short loops of Henle in rat kidney. Pflügers Arch 300: 255-282.

SCHNERMANN, J, WRIGHT, FS, DAVIS, JM, STACKELBERG, WV & GRILL, G 1970. Regulation of superficial nephron filtration rate by tubulo-glomerular feedback. Pflügers Arch 318: 147-175.

SCHOR, N, ICHIKAWA, I & BRENNER, BM 1981. Mechanisms of action of various hormones and vasoactive substancer on glomerular ultrafiltration in the rat. Kidney Int 20: 442-451.

SJÖQUIST, GÖRANSON, A, KÄLLSKOG, Ö & ULFENDAHL, HR 1984. The influence of glomerular feedback on the autoregulation of filtration rate in superficial and deep glomeruli. Acta Physiol Scand 122: 235-242.

STEFFES, MW, BUCHWALD, BD, WIGNESS, TJG, RUPP, MR, ROHDE, PJB & MAUER, SM 1982. Diabetic nephropathy in the uninephrectomized dog: Microscopic lesions after one year. Kidney Int 21: 721-724.

STEINHAUSEN, M, KUCHERER, H, PAREKH, N, WEIS, S, WIEGMAN, D L & WILHELM, K-R 1986. Angiotensin II control of the renal microcirculation: Effect of blockade by saralasin. Kidney Int 30: 56-61.

STEVEN, K 1974a. Influence of nephron GFR on proximal reabsorption In pentobarbital anesthetized rats. Kidney Int 5: 204-213.

STEVEN, K 1974b. Effect of peritubular infusion of angiotensin II on rat proximal nephron function. Kidney Int 6: 73-80.

STEVEN, K 1977. Glomerulotubular balance in the rat kidney. Acta Physiol Scand suppl 447: 1-30.

STEVEN, K AND S STRØBÆK 1974. Renal corpuscular hydrodynamics: digital computer simulation. Pflügers Arch 348: 317-331.

STUMPE, KO, LOWITZ, HD & OCHWADT, B 1970. Fluid reabsorption in Henle's loop and urinary excretion of sodium and water in normal rats and rats with chronic hypertension. J Clin Invest 49: 1200-1212.

TUCKER, BJ & BLANTZ, RC 1977. An analysis of the determinants of nephron filtration rate. Am J Physiol 232: F477-F483.

TUCKER, BJ & BLANTZ, RC 1981. Effects of glomerular filtration dynamics on the glomerular permeability coefficient. Am J Physiol 240: F245-F254.

VAN ITALIE, CM & FERNSTROM, JD 1982. Osmolal effects on vasopressin secretion in the streptozotocin-diabetic rat. Am J Physiol 242: E411-E417.

WELLING, LW & GRANTHAM, JJ 1972. Physical properties of isolated perfused renal tubules basement membranes. J Clin Invest 51: 1063-1075.

WELLING, LW & WELLING, DJ 1978. Physical properties of isolated perfused basement membrane from rabbit loop of Henle. Am J Physiol 234: F54-F58.

WELLING, LW & WELLING, DJ 1975. Pressure-flow-diameter relationship in isolated perfused thin limb of Henle. Am J Physiol 229: 1-7.

WILLIAMSON, JR, VOGLER, NJ & KILO, C 1971. Regional variation in the width of the basement membrane of muscle capillaries in man and giraffe. Am J Pathol 63: 359-367.

WRIGHT, SF 1982. Flow-dependent transport processes: filtration, absorption, secretion. Am J Physiol 243: F1-F11.

YOSHIDA, Y, FOGO, A, SHIRAGA, H, GLICK, AD & ICHIKAWA, I 1988. Serial micropuncture analysis of single nephron function in subtotal renal ablation. Kidney Int 33: 855-867.

ZATZ, R, DUNN, BR, MEYER, TW, ANDERSON, S, RENNKE, HG & BRENNER, BM 1986. Prevention of diabetic glomerulopathy by pharmacological amelioration of glomerular capillary hypertension. J Clin Invest 77: 1925-1930.

ZATZ, R, MEYER, TW, RENNKE, HG & BRENNER, BM 1985. Predominance of hemodynamic rather than metabolic factors in the pathogenesis of diabetic glomerulopathy. Proc Natl Acad Sci USA 82: 5963-5967.